Understanding
Shiatsu

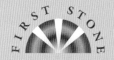

FIRST STONE

Contents

1

What is Shiatsu?

Shiatsu is a form of therapeutic bodywork that is relaxing, restorative and beneficial to health. Treatment sessions take place at floor level on a futon (padded mat) with the client wearing light, loose clothing.

Although a Shiatsu practitioner may include a range of techniques and approaches in each session, treatments can be characterised as having three main features:

- Relaxed perpendicular pressure – the practitioner will use fingers, thumbs and occasionally elbows or knees to press key points and areas in the body
- Stretching – gentle stretching of the limbs in specific directions to release or stimulate the body's energetic functions
- Mobilisation – rotations of the joints as required, again to release and relax.

THE BENEFITS
Shiatsu is a deeply relaxing experience and regular Shiatsu

sessions help to prevent the build up of stress in our daily lives.

Stress is a widely acknowledged factor of modern life. If not addressed, stress and strain, which start out affecting our emotional well-being, can end up producing physical symptoms as well. How can the physical touch therapy of Shiatsu help these stresses, which have an emotional as well as physical content, to melt away?

All the emotional stresses of daily life are stored in our body, and need to be released to

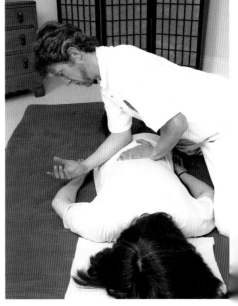

▲ Relaxed perpendicular pressure: Elbows and forearms are part of the Shiatsu 'toolkit' and can be applied effectively without causing pain.

enable us to move forward in daily life.

For example, when we are shocked by a bus passing very close to us, our whole body reacts with tension. That tension remains with the body unless it is released in some way.

Similarly, someone who habitually hunches up their shoulders and contracts their chest may have learnt, possibly from bad experiences, to close off emotionally and not open up to people. This memory pattern is stored in the body and prevents

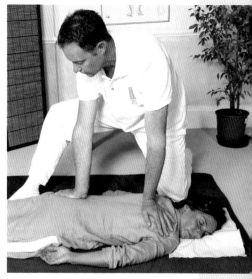

▲ *Stretching: Applying a gentle stretch to ease tension*

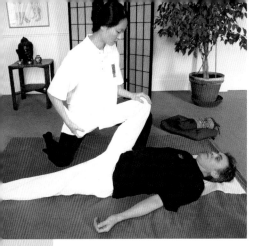

▲ *Mobilisation: Rotations and stretches help to mobilise the joints.*

In addition, the special quality of 'Shiatsu-touch', being touched in a therapeutic, non-invasive but supportive way, can by itself be very healing.

There are many benefits to Shiatsu treatment, both general and specific. Though more profound benefits will usually emerge during the course of a series of treatments, more obvious benefits will be evident from the start. These may include:

- Relaxation to mind and body
- Restoring and balancing energy

us living life to the full. Shiatsu can help, in a gentle and supportive way, to remove these blocks.

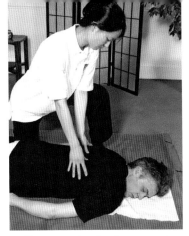

▲ *Shiatsu is a deeply relaxing experience. Here thumb pressure is being applied to the meridians of the back.*

- Easing of tension and stiffness
- Improvement to breathing
- Better posture
- Improved circulation
- Increased well-being.

WHO CAN IT HELP?

People choose Shiatsu for a variety of reasons and often, in the first instance, it is an immediate physical symptom. It may be a condition that occurred recently, such as a sports injury, or may be longer term.

On the following page we have included a list, though not an exhaustive one, of common conditions that have been helped by Shiatsu.

- Back pain
- Headaches and migraines
- Whiplash injuries and neck stiffness
- Joint pain and reduced mobility
- Menstrual problems
- Digestive problems
- Asthmatic or other breathing difficulties
- Sports injuries
- Depression.

The quality of touch in Shiatsu treatment has the effect of awakening the client's own self-healing process. If the person's energy can be balanced out and revitalized, then healing will take place.

For this reason, Shiatsu can be used to treat a wide range of complaints and chronic conditions very effectively. In this sense, Shiatsu and orthodox medicine are complementary to each other in their ability to help people.

However, as anyone who has been involved in Shiatsu for some time will tell you, these benefits are only the tip of the iceberg in terms of exploring the full potential of this therapy.

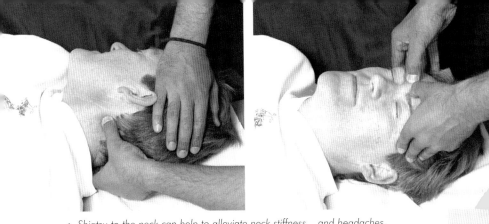

▲ *Shiatsu to the neck can help to alleviate neck stiffness... and headaches.*

As a genuinely holistic therapy, able to address the mind, emotions and spirit through physical touch, Shiatsu has become part of the lifestyle management of many busy, fulfilled individuals. Many people come for Shiatsu on a regular basis to de-stress and revitalize, leaving the treatment room feeling brighter, lighter and more cheerful.

11

2 History
of
Shiatsu

The modern development of Shiatsu in the form recognisably practised today started during the early part of the 20th century in Japan. It was at this time that the term 'Shiatsu' ('shi' meaning 'finger' and 'atsu' meaning 'pressure') was first coined.

The term 'Shiatsu' was first used by Tamai Tempaku as part of an effort to establish some scientific credibility and to distinguish Shiatsu from other forms of oriental bodywork.

Tempaku wrote two books, *Shiatsu Ryoku* (1915) and *Shiatsu Ho* (1919), in which he described the benefits of Shiatsu in western – as opposed to oriental – medical terms. He also located the acupoints by physiological terms instead of by the usual methods of traditional medicine.

DEVELOPING THE THERAPY
After Tempaku, Shiatsu developed in two different directions. One of Tempaku's students was Namikoshi, who had also studied western medicine.

He took the route of westernising Shiatsu still further, by using neuro-muscular terminology and removing any reference to concepts of oriental medicine, such as meridians and acupoints. He took his style of Shiatsu to the United States, where it is still popular.

The main style of Shiatsu in the UK and Europe was developed by Shizuto Masunaga (1925-1976), and has come to be known as Zen Shiatsu. Masunaga had a background in psychology and was able to integrate many psychological or emotional characteristics into the structure of oriental medical thought.

One of these is the concept that the attitude of mind, awareness and focus of the practitioner is an important factor in treatment. This directly affects the quality of the experience of a Shiatsu session.

Masunaga also introduced the notion of support and connection through the use of both hands, one acting as the 'mother hand' and the other as the active or working hand. This method allows the experience of Shiatsu

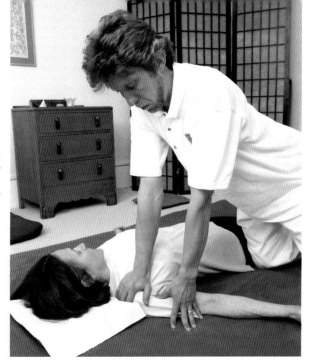

The focus ▶ and intention of the practictioner is an important factor in the effectiveness of treatment.

15

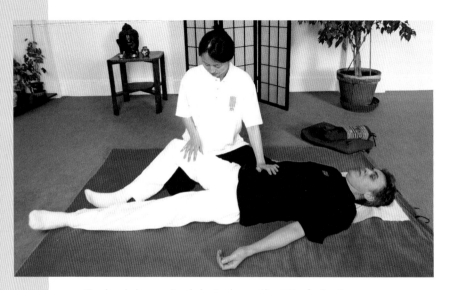

▲ *Two-handed connection helps to deepen the state of relaxation.*

to be deeper and more profound and nurturing. In addition, he developed some key concepts, which are unique to modern Shiatsu, including the extended meridian system, methods of diagnosis and approaches to treatment.

NEW INSIGHTS

The theories and approaches of Shiatsu have continued to develop since the deaths of its two main proponents. In recent years, leading practitioners have developed their own styles based on insights they have gained into the human condition through their own research and experience.

As a result, some new nomenclature has arisen, such as Ohashiatsu, Tao Shiatsu and Quantum Shiatsu.

However, it can safely be stated that all these more recent developments not only owe a huge debt to the work of Masunaga or Namikoshi, but are firmly based in the theories and practice developed by them.

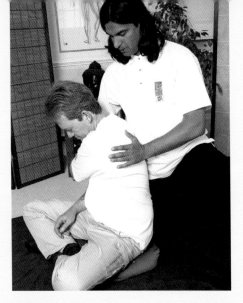

Background to Shiatsu

The underlying principles of Shiatsu are to be found deep in the history of oriental thought. For the ancient Chinese, the principles that govern human life are the same as those forces that are found to be guiding Nature and all natural processes.

This viewpoint or philosophy is understood at various levels, from the most unified and abstract to the particular, from the motions of the stars to the movement of the blood.

TAO

The most fundamental description of life is known as the Tao, which translates as The Way or Path. This is the most unified of oriental theories of life, and by definition defies description or analysis.

It is the "way" of life itself and is therefore something that has to be lived and experienced rather than talked about. This is a key point made in the *Tao Te Ching*, the definitive guide to the Tao, believed to have been written in the 6th century BC by Lao Tse.

The Tao is ever present and in

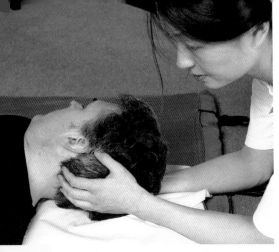

▲ *The Shiatsu practitioner seeks to maintain an awareness of the energetic interaction between giver and receiver.*

The aim of the Taoist is to live life with an emphasis on spontaneity and naturalness, with an intuitive sense of being at one with the Tao.

This has its bearing on the attitude of a Shiatsu practitioner who seeks to maintain an overall awareness of the energetic interaction between giver and receiver. In Shiatsu, it is important not to force change (or healing) but to support the creation of conditions in which change, improvement and balance can naturally take place.

itself unchanging and accomplishes everything in Nature without apparent effort.

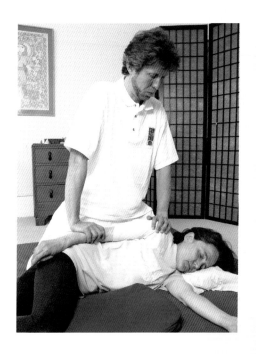

Pressure sensitively ▶ applied makes for a very satisfying and relaxing experience for the client.

As part of this, Shiatsu is done without using physical force, either to press on the body or to move it. The focus instead is on gravity and the relaxed use of body weight to achieve pressure.

Movement is a kind of dance where the practitioner uses his/her centre of balance as a fulcrum around which stretches or rotations can be carried out. This relaxed and natural feel of giving the treatment comes across to the recipient as an experience that is pleasurable and relaxing.

These are important factors in creating a genuine healing process. Changes that are forced on the body under stress, or that are sharply painful, are unlikely to be long-lasting.

YIN AND YANG

The philosophy of the Tao is further refined by the observation that everything in nature expresses two opposing (yet complementary and interdependent) forces, known as Yin and Yang.

While the Tao is essentially an understanding of creation, the Yin/Yang theory is a description of how the universe actually works in practice. Likewise, it is a cornerstone of oriental medicine and influences all diagnostic procedures.

Everything contains within it a Yin and Yang aspect; even Yin and Yang themselves, as can be seen from the symbol (opposite). Each pole contains the seed of its opposite within itself. The simplest delineation of Yin and Yang is perhaps night and day. We can see, even at one minute past midnight, that the day and

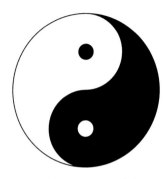

▲ *The Yin/Yang symbol*

originally meant 'the shady side of a slope', and Yin is associated with cold, rest, passivity, darkness, inwardness and decrease.

Yang, the sunny side of the slope, is associated with heat, stimulation, movement, activity, excitement, vigour, light, expansion and increase.

It is important not to apply moral values to Yin and Yang, in the sense that either one is better than the other. Both are ever present, their rise and fall is a function of the changing nature of life and both are equally necessary.

the dawn are already on their way. Yang is more masculine than feminine, yet everyone has both Yin (feminine) and Yang (masculine) within them.

The Chinese character for Yin

23

In oriental medicine, the meridians (see below) and their associated organs have been paired according to their Yin or Yang characteristics.

The Yin and Yang qualities of the human body have been further divided into four pairs and form an important baseline of diagnosis in oriental medicine, known as the Eight Principles.

The four pairs are:
- Interior/exterior
- Hot/cold
- Full/empty
- Yin and Yang (which serve to summarise and coalesce the other symptoms).

This is already a useful method of diagnosis by identifying symptoms as showing an excess or deficiency within the Eight Principles. For example, a fever shows symptoms of excess heat. To regulate the body, and bring a return to homoeostasis, it is necessary to cool the person down. So we naturally encourage the patient to drink cool fluids and to apply moist cloths to reduce the fever.

THE YIN ORGANS

Spleen

Lungs

Liver

Heart

Heart protector

Kidneys

These are seen as more Yin because of their supportive role in "storing precious substance" with qualities of nourishing, cooling and moistening.

THE YANG ORGANS

Stomach

Large intestine

Gall bladder

Small intestine

Triple heater

Bladder

These organs have more energetic, moving functions and are concerned with the energy supplying the organs.

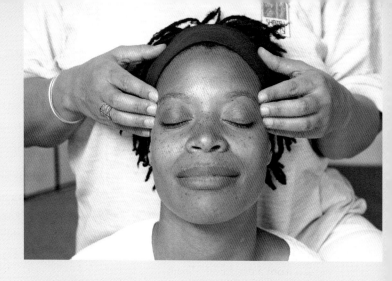

4 Principles of Shiatsu

The main working principle underlying Shiatsu is that the human organism, and indeed all life forms, is vitalized by different types, quantities and qualities of Ki (energy).

KI

At its most fundamental level, Ki is our basic life force and distinguishes, for example, a live person from a dead body. From the point of view of oriental thought, Ki is as much an aspect of physical life as blood and bone.

One way of looking at it is to see Ki as providing the driving force to the body's functions, such as the pumping of blood around the body or the action of the lymph or digestive system.

From this, we can gain an idea of the quality or strength of an individual's Ki, and see it manifesting in robust good health or in illness or lack of energy. "I'm feeling tired today" or "I feel really well and optimistic" can be seen as descriptions of how Ki is functioning in us at any particular time.

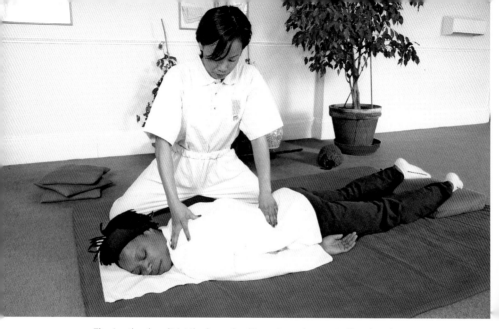

▲ *The 'mother hand' (at the lower back) monitors changes in Ki induced by the working hand.*

At all times, we are exchanging Ki with our environment, through breathing, eating, walking, talking, etc. From this point of view, it is obvious that eating good-quality foods, high in their Ki level, getting plenty of fresh air to increase our intake of Ki, and adequate rest, to restore our Ki, are fundamentally important in maintaining health.

MERIDIANS

The Shiatsu practitioner works directly with an individual's Ki in a treatment through the main network of 'Ki carriers' in the body, known as meridians. One of the main aims of a Shiatsu practitioner's training is to develop sensitivity to the movement and condition of Ki in the recipient.

In an ideal situation, an individual's Ki will flow unimpeded and with great vitality through all the meridians. For many different reasons Ki can stop flowing freely, and this then produces a symptom. There is an old saying: where there is free flow of Ki, there is no pain. Reactions to a weak or impeded flow of Ki can include anything from a feeling of sluggishness to a clinically defined condition.

The flow of Ki through the meridians can be imagined as a network of rivers. A healthy person's meridians can be understood as rivers flowing in an even, unobstructed way, whereas an unhealthy person's meridians can be seen as rivers where there are blockages, places where there is too much or too little water, or even where the course of the river has been diverted underground.

Strung along the meridians are the acupoints, the same as those which will be needled by an acupuncturist. As a result of many hundreds of years of empirical study, these points have been found to have certain actions and functions in affecting a person's energy and overall health.

The actions are usually closely linked to the qualities of the meridian as well as to the oriental understanding of the causes of disease.

The study of acupoints and their related Zang Fu (the study

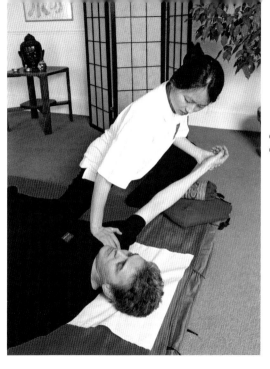

◄ Gentle stretching opens the meridian and eases the joints.

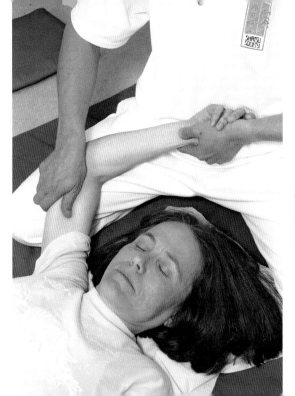

◄ The practictioner will move the client's limbs to improve access to specific meridians.

of the organs) is known as TCM (Traditional Chinese Medicine) to distinguish it from Five Element Theory (below).

The Shiatsu practitioner's focus in a treatment is primarily to rebalance and regulate the flow of Ki in the client. The effect of therapeutic touch, which affects the muscles, blood and bones of the recipient, is to improve the flow of Ki and to bring about an improved state of health.

FIVE ELEMENTS

As mentioned earlier, Shiatsu is a great therapy for stress or lifestyle management because treatment also reaches the emotional, mental and spiritual aspects of our lives.

Five Element Theory brings together the way in which the physical body integrates with emotional, mental and spiritual aspects. Since each meridian is an expression of one of the Five Elements (Water, Wood, Fire, Earth and Metal), Shiatsu treatment can directly benefit all aspects of ourselves and, as such, is a genuinely holistic therapy.

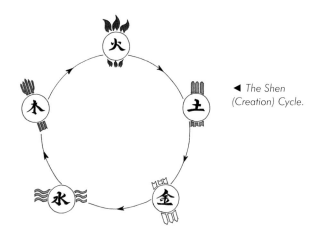

◄ The Shen
(Creation) Cycle.

The Five Elements, or more accurately translated the Five Phases, apply not only to humans but are also a way of describing nature itself, of which humans are a part. Therefore, the same principles that apply in Nature itself are observed in us.

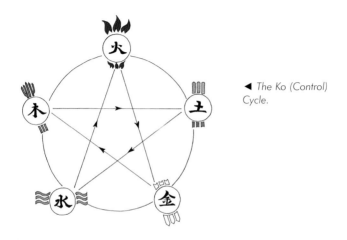

◄ The Ko (Control) Cycle.

These phases, defined as Water, Wood, Fire, Earth and Metal, describe the changing rhythms in nature, and can therefore be applied to any field of human endeavour, such as philosophy, agriculture, nutrition, etc., as well as

35

ELEMENT	Water	Wood	Fire	Earth	Metal
MERIDIANS	Kidney Bladder	Liver Gall bladder	Heart Small intestine Heart protector Triple heater	Spleen Stomach	Lung Large intestine
Voice	Groan	Shout	Laugh	Sing	Weep
Emotions	Fear	Anger	Joy	Thought	Grief
Physical	Bones	Sinews	Blood	Muscles	Skin
Colour	Blue/black	Green	Red	Yellow	White
Taste	Salt	Sour	Bitter	Sweet	Pungent
Season	Winter	Spring	Summer	Late summer	Autumn

◄ A selection of the correspondences, including the meridians associated with each one.

medicine. At their most general and easily understood, the Five Elements describe the pattern of the seasons: winter (Water), spring (Wood), summer (Fire) and autumn (Metal). This natural sequence is shown on page 34 and is known as the Shen or Creation Cycle.

The Earth element is usually described as late summer, after Fire, as that lingering harvest period. However, since the earth underpins all other life forms and activities, the Earth element can also be seen as being continuously present

37

during the cycle of the seasons. This cycle is also known as the Mother-Child cycle since each phase gives birth to the next.

In addition there is a second cycle, the Ko or Control Cycle, which has a more active and dynamic interaction (see page 35). As opposed to the apparently orderly procession through the seasons as seen in the Shen Cycle, we have the image of a more Yang transformation of the Elements, which we can picture as: Metal cuts Wood, Fire burns or melts Metal, Wood breaks through the Earth, and the Earth guides Water in channels.

Within us, the Five Elements are seen in our emotions, facial hue, the quality of our voice, preferred taste, etc.

The table on page 36 shows a selection of the correspondences, including the meridians associated with each one.

It is important to note that the diagnostic features of these are apparent only when there is imbalance or disharmony in a certain element. For example, there are people who always seem to be shouting, even when talking normally in an ordinary conversation. One could conclude from this that their Wood Element may be somewhat out of balance. And when someone has a streaming cold, their face will tend to be a bright white colour, indicating that their Metal element, specifically the Lung meridian, is struggling for equilibrium.

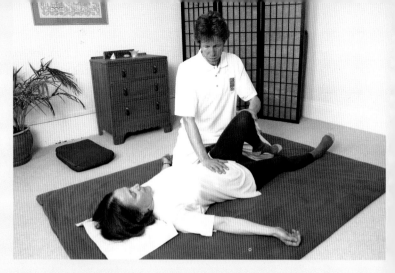

5

A Shiatsu Treatment

The theories of oriental medicine, as previously outlined, form the background to a diagnostic understanding of the receiver's condition. The main traditional methods of diagnosis are classified as looking, listening (and smelling), asking questions and touch.

SHIATSU DIAGNOSIS

From the moment the client enters the room, the practitioner will be able to start building up a picture. The colour of the face, for example, as shown in the table on page 36, may give an overall impression according to the Five Elements.

In addition, each part of the face is associated with a meridian, and any discoloration, swelling or any other sign may indicate an imbalance within its associated channel or Element.

The tone of voice will also give diagnostic information. With a little practice, especially with the eyes closed, it is possible to discern the different tones, such as groaning, shouting, etc., that will indicate a possible imbalance in one Element or another.

Often, a person's voice will carry more than one tone in a layered effect, which again may be useful information.

Questioning, in addition to conversational inquiry, will usually take the form of a written case history where information about a client's medical history, aches and pains, sleep patterns, dietary preferences and other aspects will be gathered.

At the first session, this is discussed in some detail. The practitioner identifies the reasons why someone has come for Shiatsu and what they will hope to achieve through a treatment or series of treatments.

TOUCH DIAGNOSIS

As one might expect from a touch-based therapy, the touch itself is the most important and significant diagnostic tool.

While the other methods of diagnosis outlined above are

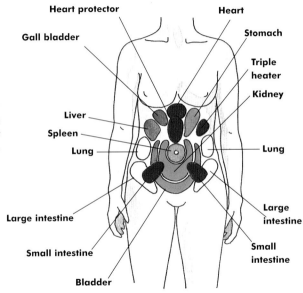

Heart protector

Heart

Gall bladder

Stomach

Triple heater

Kidney

An illustration ▶ of the abdomen (Hara) diagnostic areas.

Liver

Spleen

Lung

Lung

Large intestine

Large intestine

Small intestine

Small intestine

Bladder

43

important, when it comes to the actual Shiatsu treatment, it is the information gained through touch diagnosis that will be used to guide the type and level of the treatment itself.

Information gained through other methods will be held as background and, as a general rule, will not influence the treatment directly. That said, practitioners who work more with the TCM functions of acupoints may place more emphasis on the effect of points to treat prevailing conditions that have shown up in the preliminary forms of diagnosis.

The distinguishing mark of Shiatsu diagnosis is the palpation for the Kyo (empty or hidden) and Jitsu (full or overactive) condition of the meridians. This is carried out through lightly touching the diagnostic areas of the Hara (abdomen) that relate to each meridian (see page 43).

This unique form of diagnosis, developed by Masunaga, gives the practitioner information of the immediate energetic situation of the client on which

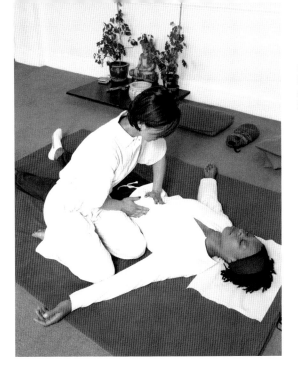

◀ The abdomen (Hara) is an important diagnostic area in Shiatsu.

to base the treatment.

It is a truism to say that you cannot treat yesterday's or tomorrow's energy, and the Hara diagnosis creates the opportunity to work right in the present on what the client is presenting at the time.

WHAT HAPPENS

The session then takes place at floor level on a futon. Shiatsu in a therapeutic context is carried out with the client lying on his/her back, front or side.

Within each treatment, at least two, if not all three,

positions will tend to be used. The practitioner may ask the client to move position each time, or may assist in helping him/her to move.

Shiatsu can also be received in a sitting position, either kneeling on the floor or sitting on a chair. However, the sitting position is not often used. Although it is an excellent way of working, moving the client on to then off a chair may break the atmosphere or rhythm created during a session.

The practitioner may, however, decide that sitting is

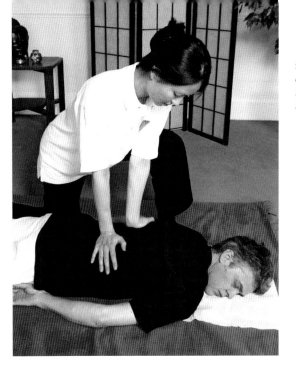

◀ Treatment can take place in different positions. Here, the back is being palmed.

47

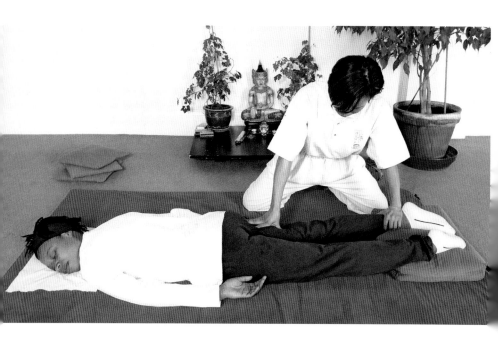

the best position to carry out a certain manoeuvre that may be more difficult in one of the other positions. It may also be preferred if the client has difficulty getting down on to the futon.

The sitting position is most often used at exhibitions and demonstrations of Shiatsu as an indicator of what is involved.

◄ *On the front: Relaxing and invigorating the legs in prone position.*

WHAT TO EXPECT

Each session lasts approximately one hour, with the treatment itself taking about 45 minutes. The first session will usually be slightly longer to include time for the initial case history.

An experienced practitioner will be sensitive to your constitution and general energy levels when selecting techniques and assessing the amount of pressure to apply.

Treatment will incorporate a variety of techniques to improve your energy flow. These may include gentle holding, pressing

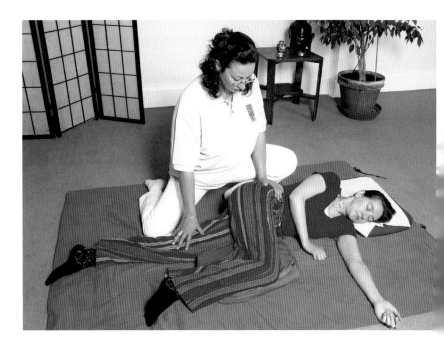

◄ Shiatsu treatment in the side position.

A range of ► stretching and movement techniques can be applied in the kneeling position.

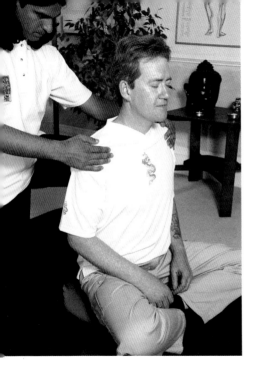

with palms, thumbs, fingers, elbows, knees and feet on the meridians and, when appropriate, more dynamic rotations and stretches.

The treatment itself should not be painful. Occasionally there may be some discomfort due to a particularly sensitive area being contacted, but this is usually experienced as a 'good' pain: in other words, the sensation feels as if it is still

◄ *Techniques for increasing flexibility and relieving tension in the back can be applied in the sitting position.*

Shiatsu is a ▶
whole-body
treatment, which
includes the
hands...

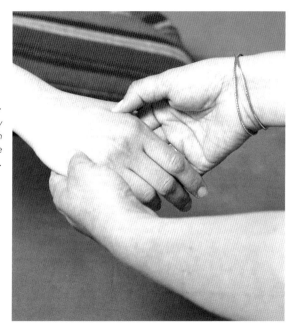

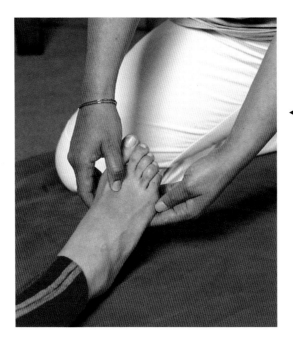

◀ ...and the feet.

beneficial in the sense of removing restrictions.

As the quality of Ki changes, the symptoms associated with a lack of flow will gradually improve. Shiatsu is a therapy that works on the individual as a complete being. It doesn't just concentrate on the physical body, but also works on an emotional and/or mental level.

This is generally experienced as a sense of deep relaxation and connectedness during the treatment, which may last for several hours or even days afterwards. Generally one feels invigorated yet relaxed.

Occasionally, and it should be emphasised that this is rare, there may be a healing reaction in the 24 to 48 hours following treatment – experienced as pain for a short while or even an emotional release through tears.

This can happen as the body's energy starts to realign towards a more balanced state; as that process takes place, a symptom appears.

It is, however, usually nothing to worry about and does not last very long.

GUIDELINES FOR TREATMENT

- Wear loose, warm, comfortable clothing, preferably cotton, e.g. sweatshirt, tracksuit trousers and cotton socks.
- Do not eat heavily in the two hours prior to treatment.
- Do not drink alcohol before or after treatment.
- After treatment drink plenty of water to smooth the flow of changes through the system.
- If at all possible, avoid strenuous or stressful activities after your session.

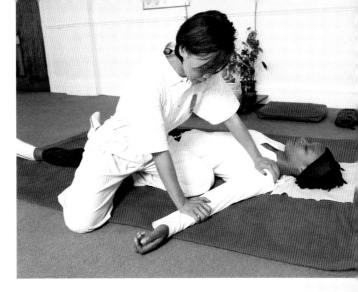

Wear loose, ▶
comfortable clothing
for your treatment.

Where To Find Us

As with any therapeutic treatment, it is important to find a Shiatsu practitioner who is suitably qualified and a member of a professional organisation. The best way to find a qualified practitioner near you is through the Shiatsu Society, which maintains two public registers of qualified practitioners:

- MRSS: Members of the professional Register of the Shiatsu Society (MRSS) have been assessed for professionalism and clinical expertise by an independent panel of senior practitioners and teachers of Shiatsu.
- Graduate: Members on the Graduate listing hold diplomas from the Society's recognised schools following three years of training, but have not yet taken (or

passed) the independent MRSS assessment.

Members of both Registers are:
- Current professional members of the Society
- Covered by professional indemnity insurance to a level set by the Society
- Provide a signed agreement to abide by the Society's Codes of Ethics and Conduct.

Names of MRSS and Graduate practitioners are available from the Society's office and website.

TRAINING IN SHIATSU

The Shiatsu Society can also provide a list of recognised schools. These offer full training in Shiatsu – from introductory courses lasting a weekend or two, up to full practitioner training.

The full training in Shiatsu takes three years, and includes modules in anatomy, physiology and pathology. Following graduation, practitioners are encouraged to come forward for assessment to join the Society's full registration as MRSS.

The Shiatsu Society (UK)

The Society was set up in 1981 to facilitate communication within the field of Shiatsu and to inform the public of the benefits of this form of natural healing. Since then, the Society has grown to form a network linking interested individuals, students and teachers, and to fulfil the role of Professional Association for Shiatsu Practitioners.

For details of training in Shiatsu or to obtain a list of MRSS and Graduate Practitioners by area, please contact:

The Shiatsu Society (UK)
Eastlands Court
St Peters Road
Rugby CV21 3QP
Tel: 0845 130 4560
Fax: 01788 555052
Email: admin@shiatsu.org
Website: www.shiatsu.org

Further Reading

Shiatsu: The Complete Guide
Chris Jarmey and Gabriel Mojay.
Thorsons, 1999
ISBN 0 7225 3914 2

Shiatsu Theory and Practice
Carola Beresford Cooke.
Churchill Livingstone, 2002
ISBN 0 443 07059 8

*The New Book of Shiatsu: Vitality
and health through the
art of touch*
Paul Lundberg.
Gaia, 2002
ISBN 1 85675 114 7

About the author

Ian Macwhinnie is a registered Shiatsu practitioner (MRSS) who has a practice in Leamington Spa, Warwickshire. He is also the Administration Manager of the Shiatsu Society (UK).

He is the author of *The Radiant Kingdom: An allegorical study of meditation* (California: Celestial Arts, 1996).

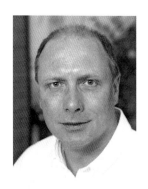

Other titles in the series

- **Understanding Acupressure**
- **Understanding Acupuncture**
- **Understanding The Alexander Technique**
- **Understanding Aromatherapy**
- **Understanding Bach Flower Remedies**
- **Understanding Echinacea**
- **Understanding Evening Primrose**
- **Understanding Feng Shui**
- **Understanding Fish Oils**
- **Understanding Garlic**
- **Understanding Ginseng**
- **Understanding Head Massage**
- **Understanding Kinesiology**
- **Understanding Lavender**
- **Understanding Massage**
- **Understanding Pilates**
- **Understanding Reflexology**
- **Understanding Reiki**
- **Understanding St. John's Wort**
- **Understanding Yoga**

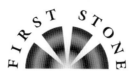

First published 2003 by First Stone Publishing
4/5 The Marina, Harbour Road, Lydney, Gloucestershire, GL15 5ET

The contents of this book are for information only and are not intended as a substitute for appropriate medical attention. The author and publishers admit no liability for any consequences arising from following any advice contained within this book. If you have any concerns about your health or medication, always consult your doctor.

Note: Capital letters have been used for foreign words as well as English words which have an extended specific meaning within the context of oriental medicine.

ISBN 1 904439 10 1
Printed and bound in Hong Kong through Printworks International Ltd.

All photographs © The Shiatsu Society (UK)